Dimiter Hadjiev

Blood Pressure Management in Stroke and in Elderly Hypertensives

Dimiter Hadjiev

Blood Pressure Management in Stroke and in Elderly Hypertensives

Blood Pressure Management in Acute Ischemic Stroke and in Elderly Hypertensive Patients

LAP LAMBERT Academic Publishing

Impressum / Imprint

Bibliografische Information der Deutschen Nationalbibliothek: Die Deutsche Nationalbibliothek verzeichnet diese Publikation in der Deutschen Nationalbibliografie; detaillierte bibliografische Daten sind im Internet über http://dnb.d-nb.de abrufbar.

Alle in diesem Buch genannten Marken und Produktnamen unterliegen warenzeichen-, marken- oder patentrechtlichem Schutz bzw. sind Warenzeichen oder eingetragene Warenzeichen der jeweiligen Inhaber. Die Wiedergabe von Marken, Produktnamen, Gebrauchsnamen, Handelsnamen, Warenbezeichnungen u.s.w. in diesem Werk berechtigt auch ohne besondere Kennzeichnung nicht zu der Annahme, dass solche Namen im Sinne der Warenzeichen- und Markenschutzgesetzgebung als frei zu betrachten wären und daher von jedermann benutzt werden dürften.

Bibliographic information published by the Deutsche Nationalbibliothek: The Deutsche Nationalbibliothek lists this publication in the Deutsche Nationalbibliografie; detailed bibliographic data are available in the Internet at http://dnb.d-nb.de.

Any brand names and product names mentioned in this book are subject to trademark, brand or patent protection and are trademarks or registered trademarks of their respective holders. The use of brand names, product names, common names, trade names, product descriptions etc. even without a particular marking in this works is in no way to be construed to mean that such names may be regarded as unrestricted in respect of trademark and brand protection legislation and could thus be used by anyone.

Coverbild / Cover image: www.ingimage.com

Verlag / Publisher:
LAP LAMBERT Academic Publishing
ist ein Imprint der / is a trademark of
OmniScriptum GmbH & Co. KG
Heinrich-Böcking-Str. 6-8, 66121 Saarbrücken, Deutschland / Germany
Email: info@lap-publishing.com

Herstellung: siehe letzte Seite /
Printed at: see last page
ISBN: 978-3-659-52473-8

Contents

Preface

Chapter 1. Blood Pressure Management in Acute Ischemic Stroke

Chapter 2. Blood Pressure Management and Cognitive Functions in Elderly Hypertensive Patients

Preface

Hypertension is the major modifiable risk factor for stroke and stroke mortality. It is also the most important risk factor for vascular cognitive impairment and vascular dementia in elderly hypertensive patients without a history of stroke. Several clinical and epidemiological studies have shown that the antihypertensive treatment reduces the stroke morbidity and mortality. However, the management of blood pressure in definite medical conditions, such as acute ischemic stroke and elderly hypertensive persons at risk of cognitive impairment remains problematic.

A transient elevated arterial blood pressure is common in acute ischemic stroke and is often associated with a poor prognosis. The underlying mechanisms of blood pressure elevation are not well understood and its management is still unresolved. There is evidence that the main causes of a transient blood pressure elevation in acute ischemic stroke are the focal cerebral hypoperfusion and the stress responses with neuroendocrine systems activation. Clinical trials have reported that blood pressure lowering in acute ischemic stroke may have detrimental effect, probably because of impaired cerebral autoregulation. However, quantitative assessment of cerebral perfusion has not been performed during emergency blood pressure reduction in acute ischemic stroke. The ultrasound carotid artery disease evaluation, and cerebral hemodynamics monitoring using bedside bilateral transcranial ultrasonography, during emergency blood pressure management in acute ischemic stroke might contribute to maintaining of an adequate penumbral perfusion and prevent infarct enlargement Such an approach could individualize the antihypertensive management in acute ischemic stroke and improve functional outcome.

Several longitudinal population epidemiological studies have shown an association between hypertension and cognition. However, the role of the antihypertensive therapy in preventing cognitive disorders in elderly hypertensive patients without a history of stroke is still a matter of debate. Cerebral white matter lesions, caused by small vessel disease and cerebral hypoperfusion, have been found in the majority of elderly hypertensive persons. They correlate with cognitive disorders, particularly impairments of attention and executive functions, while memory is relatively preserved. Excessive blood pressure lowering in elderly patients with long-standing hypertension below a certain critical level, may increase the risk of further cerebral hypoperfusion because of disrupted cerebral blood flow autoregulation. As a result, worsening of the cognitive functions could occur, especially in cases with additional vascular risk factors. It should be taken into account that hypertension is frequently accompanied by other risk factors, which may also contribute to development of vascular cognitive impairment and vascular dementia.

Five randomized, placebo-controlled trials have focused on the efficacy of antihypertensive treatments in preventing cognitive impairments in elderly hypertensive patients without a prior cerebrovascular disease. Four of them have not found positive effects. Probably, the repeated neuropsychological assessments and ultrasonography for evaluation of carotid atherosclerosis, as well as cerebral hemodynamics monitoring could adjust the antihypertensive therapy with the aim to decrease the risk of further cerebral hypoperfusion and prevent or slow down cognitive decline in elderly hypertensive patients.

The increased risk of white matter lesions in long-standing hypertension is an indication for early neuroprotection. The combination of renin-angiotensin blockade or calcium channel blockers with statins may become a promising preventive strategy against cognitive decline in elderly hypertensive persons. Mediterranean diet is also thought to possess a beneficial effect on cognitive functions. Cerebral white matter protection is a future challenge.

Obviously, blood pressure management in acute ischemic stroke and in elderly hypertensives at risk for cognitive decline must be carefully controlled. The clinical criteria and impaired cerebral autoregulation should be considered when administering antihypertensive treatment. Transcranial Doppler ultrasonography proved to be an useful method in the assessment of cerebral hemodynamics and the effects of different antihypertensive drugs. This method could become a valuable tool to monitor cerebral hemodynamic changes in acute stroke patients and in elderly hypertensive patients with the aim to individualize the antihypertensive treatment.

Neuroprotection in acute stroke and in elderly hypertensive patients at high risk for cognitive impairment, until evidence-based data are not available, remains a challenge to future well designed studies.

Chapter 1.

Blood Pressure Management in Acute Ischemic Stroke

Introduction

Several studies have shown that the transient elevated arterial blood pressure (BP) in acute ischemic stroke (IS) is a very frequent finding and is often associated with a poor outcome. High BP levels with a marked spontaneous decline have been found in acute stroke patients after emergency hospital admission. The highest values of BP have been recorded in previously hypertensive persons and the higher the initial BP the greater the decline [1–3]. High BP, measured at a median time of 20 hours after symptom onset has been found in about 80% of the patients with acute IS. A U-shaped relationship has been observed between baseline SBP and both early death and late death or dependency [4].

However, the reason for the transient BP elevation is still debatable [6]. Besides, the appropriate treatment of arterial hypertension in acute IS is not yet settled and the results of the present clinical trials are controversial. BP management in the setting of acute IS remains problematic and the questions such as when to start antihypertensives and by how much to reduce BP are not yet resolved [7,8].

A large body of trials have tested the effects of different vasoactive drugs in acute IS, but the available data do not allow the effect of changing BP on IS outcome to be assessed [9–10]. That is why the recommended levels of BP lowering in acute IS are still based on panel consensus [7]. It could also be pointed out that the clinical trials on the efficacy of different antihypertensive drugs in acute IS have several limitations. They have often included patients with both ischemic and hemorrhagic strokes [11]. Although it has been shown that some antihypertensive drugs may cause an excessive fall in cerebral blood flow (CBF) [12], the cerebral hemodynamics has not been monitored in acute IS. Besides, stenoses or occlusions of the internal carotid or vertebral arteries have not been taken into consideration when antihypertensive therapy in acute IS is administered.

Undoubtedly, the appropriate BP management in patients with acute IS is of a great importance for functional outcome. It could be supposed that the BP lowering in the setting of acute IS may lead to infarct enlargement with consequent more severe neurological symptoms and cognitive dysfunction. However, this issue is still unresolved.

Pathophysiology of blood pressure elevation in acute ischemic stroke
The elevated BP in acute IS usually decreases spontaneously in the next few days of admission without antihypertensive therapy [1,2]. The pathophysiology of the transient elevated BP in acute IS is complex and not well understood. Different mechanisms have been suggested to explain BP elevation and its spontaneous decrease in acute IS. Previous hypertension has been shown to be the strongest predictor of elevated BP on admission to the hospital [1,2,13].

Carlberg et al.[13] propose that the elevated BP in patients with acute IS could be a result from the mental stress on hospital admission. The acute mental stress may be a major contributor to high BP on hospital admission, and the emergency room setting in particular, in acute stroke patients. It has been suggested that the marked spontaneous BP decline in acute IS might be caused by the stress diminishing, due to the patient's adaptation to disease and environment.

6

High plasma cortisol and catecholamines have been found in patients with acute IS. It has been pointed out that the high plasma norepinephrine in stroke patients is consistent with an increased in peripheral sympathetic activity, which could produce cardiac arrhythmias, ECG abnormalities and raised serum cardiac enzymes. The mean cortisol concentration in patients with acute IS has been also elevated, possibly via hypothalamic mechanisms, although stress could not completely be excluded [14]. It has been suggested that the hypercortisolism may be a result of repeated stresses, experienced by stroke patients [15]. The repeated stresses, which are common for stroke patients may cause abnormalities in the cortisol axis, both at the central level and at the adrenal level, and therefore prolong the hypercortisolism. Many patients with acute stroke show a pronounced hypercortisolism [16]. The early activation of the sympathetic adrenomedullar pathways may increase the risk of death in acute IS patients [17].

In a clinicopathological study a relationship between acute BP evaluation in stroke patients and the side of the brain lesion has been observed. Lesions in the caudal brain stem, especially the pons, play a role in BP elevation following cerebrovascular accidents. In primary pontine lesion a prominent pressor reaction occurred. The pressor response is more remarkable with tegmental pontine lesions, than when the lesion is in the basilar pons. It is suggested that the pressor reaction following pontine vascular lesions could originate in some inherent functions of the pons, but medulla oblongata may be also involved [18].

Another study has shown that the ventromedial prefrontal cortex lesions may increase the sympathetic hyperexcitability, resulting in anxiety, hypertension or cardiac arrhythmias [19]. It is suggested that the damage or compression of these

7

specific brain regions is the primary cause of the acute hypertensive response in acute stroke. Increased sympathoadrenal tone with subsequent release of renin and vasoconstriction of arterioles leads to an elevation of BP. Hypertensive responses could be also result from parasympathetic activity and baroreceptor sensitivity [6]. However, the spontaneous decline of the elevated BP in acute IS could not be explained by the permanent damage of the brain areas, involved in the BP regulation. Probably, these damages are transient, associated with brain edema and increased intracranial pressure.

The transient BP elevation in acute IS could also be a response to the decreased focal cerebral perfusion. In patients with acute IS treated with thrombolysis, a decrease in the systolic blood pressure (SBP) has been found when recanalization succeeded, but it remains elevated longer time when recanalization fails. The elevated SBP at admission shows a downward course in the following hours, which is accelerated by recanalization and recanalization increases the chances of favorable outcome [20]. These data suggest that the transient BP elevation is associated with focal brain ischemia, followed by activation of the sympathetic nervous system and mental stress. Spontaneous BP decline could be explained by restoration of the collateral blood circulation or successful revascularization.

Evidently, the mechanisms of the transient elevated BP in patients with acute IS are complex and should be carefully analyzed with aim to individualize the treatment approaches and prevent poor functional outcome.

Management of blood pressure elevation in acute ischemic stroke
Although, a large body of clinical trials have been completed [10], the dilemma not to treat [21] or to treat [22] elevated BP in acute IS is still unresolved. However, it

8

is pointed out when BP is badly managed to the point that cerebral perfusion falls off the left end of the autoregulation curve, CBF is reduced [22].

Neurological worsening after diastolic blood pressure (DBP) reduction is observed in patients with acute IS (within 24 hours), receiving high-dose intravenous nimodipine. Patients with a DBP reduction of >20% have a significantly increased risk of death or dependency 21 days after symptom onset. In the low-dose nimodipine group or placebo neurological worsening has no been observed. It is suggested that the profound hypotension in patients with acute IS and altered CBF autoregulation may cause a further reduction in the cerebral perfusion pressure and a decrease in regional CBF below the lethal thresholds in the penumbra [23].

Another trial has also reported that in a series of consecutive and non selected patients with acute IS, the early administration of antihypertensive drugs and a fall in SBP more than 20 mmHg during the first days after admission is associated with early neurological deterioration and a poor outcome. A U-shaped relationship between BP levels and outcome measures has been observed. The lowest frequency of a poor prognosis has been found at approximately 180 mmHg for SBP. These findings indicate that the use of antihypertensive agents and the fall in BP during the first days after admission are detrimental for patients with acute IS. It is suggested that the spontaneous BP decrease in the first days after stroke onset or other causes of fall in BP that are not controlled may contribute to the poor outcome [24].

Recently, a large randomized, placebo-controlled, double-blind trial, including 2029 patients with SBP of 140 mmHg or higher within 30 h of symptom onset has been completed. The functional outcome at the 6 months has been measured by the modified Rankin Scale. The trial has shown that the BP lowering with the angiotensin-receptor blocker, candesartan is not beneficial in patients with acute stroke and raised BP. Furthermore, treatment with candesartan has probably been associated with an increased risk of a poor functional outcome compared with placebo. It is pointed out that the routine BP lowering treatment in patients with acute stroke and raised BP could not be recommended [11].

It is important to note that in the clinical trials on the BP management in acute IS the following-up period is short, no more than 6 months, and the cognitive functions have not been taken into consideration. In such a way the long-term outcomes remain unknown.

Few studies have focused on the cerebral perfusion in the course of antihypertensive treatment in patients with acute IS. A small randomized trial has shown that nicardipine administered in previously hypertensive patients with acute IS may cause an excessive fall in BP and impair CBF, measured by single photon emission computed tomography (SPECT) [12]. In acute IS patients the severity of SPECT graded scale on the admission, within 6 hours of symptom onset, has been found to be positively associated with poor long-term outcome. It is pointed out that the measurement of an ischemic deficit using cerebral SPECT may be useful for selecting patients in clinical trials and could impact acute management decisions [25].

CBF autoregulation in acute IS patients has been studied, using bedside transcranial Doppler ultrasonography (TDS). An impaired dynamic, but not static, cerebral autoregulation has been found after the stroke onset, which remains abnormal for at least 1-2 weeks post ictus. The reduction of systematic BP may cause a decrease in cerebral perfusion pressure resulting from altered CBF autoregulation. The antihypertensive treatment in acute IS could be potentially harmful by increasing the size of the ischemic penumbra with a reduction in systematic BP levels. It is pointed out that TDS is the only method that allows to study the dynamic changes in CBF autoregulation, because of the necessary time resolution [26]. Evidently, testing the dynamic cerebral autoregulation by TDS could be a promising tool to assess the risk of brain hypoperfusion, especially in elderly hypertensive patients.

Another small study in patients, 1 to 11 days after hemispheric IS, using positron emission tomography (PET), has found in some cases a reduction of the CBF in both hemispheres after intravenous nicardipine and mean arterial pressure (MAP) lowering. It is pointed out that the individual monitoring of change in global CBF, such as with bedside TDS, may be useful to determine individual safe limit when BP is lowering in the setting of acute IS [27].

A systematic review of clinical controlled trials that have assessed the effects of antihypertensive agents on CBF and flow velocity in acute IS has found few quality studies on this topic. Several small randomized trials have assessed CBF with various antihypertensive agents in acute IS and have not shown a change in cerebral perfusion. However, there are no large randomized trials assessing outcome with BP lowering in acute stroke [28]. Obviously, further well-designed studies on quantitative assessment of CBF are needed to evaluate the effects of the antihypertensive drugs on cerebral perfusion in acute IS.

Further consideration requires the BP lowering in acute IS patients with severe carotid disease. Occlusion or severe stenosis of internal carotid artery, more than 70%, affects cerebral metabolism, assessed by magnetic resonance spectroscopic imaging, in the ipsilateral hemisphere. The metabolic changes are reflected in a decreased N-acetyl aspartate / choline ratio and a high incidence of cerebral lactate. These regions of altered cerebral metabolism are at increased risk for infarction if the cerebral perfusion pressure is declined further [29]. An increased oxygen extraction, measured by PET, distal to symptomatic carotid artery occlusion has been shown an independent risk factor for subsequent stroke [30].

An impaired cerebrovascular reactivity, using TDS, has been documented in patients with carotid occlusion, associated with an increased risk of cerebral ischemic events [31]. In patients with severe bilateral carotid artery stenosis, 70% or more, a negative correlation between BP level and risk of stroke has been found, suggesting that aggressive BP lowering may not be safe in these cases. However, no data on the presence or severity of carotid disease have been recorded in the trials of BP lowering after stroke or transient ischemic attack (TIA). It is pointed out that more data are required on the effects of BP lowering on cerebral perfusion in patients with severe bilateral carotid artery stenosis and guidelines on treatment of hypertension should highlight the need for special consideration [32]. However, only one ongoing randomized controlled trial on the efficacy of BP lowering in acute IS has included patients with significant ipsilateral carotid artery stenosis. An interim assessment has suggested that the functional outcome, evaluated by modified Rankin scale, after 90 days has been worse in patients with a baseline carotid artery stenosis 50% or more [33].

Obviously, the main variable that should be measured and monitored during antihypertensive treatment in acute IS is the cerebral hemodynamics. The decrease in CBF under certain level, because of impaired CBF autoregulation [34], could worsen the focal cerebral perfusion and enlarge the infarct size with consequent poor outcomes.

Although no data from controlled clinical trials are available, guidelines suggest that for patients not receiving intravenous thrombolytic treatment, the emergency administration of antihypertensive agents should be withheld unless the DBP is > 120 mmHg or SBP > 220 mmHg. BP lowering should be done cautiously and a reasonable goal would be by 15% to 25% within the first day. In patients undergoing thrombolysis SPB above 185 mmHg should be avoided [7, 35].

In addition, in many centers BP reduction is only considered in the presence of severe cardiac insufficiency, acute renal failure, aortic arch dissection or malignant hypertension [35]. However, in these cases the cerebral hemodynamics is not considered.

Discussion

An elevated BP is present in about 80% of the patients with acute IS and in the next few days it often declines spontaneously [1, 2]. Several studies have shown that the elevated BP in acute IS is associated with a poor outcome. Another large study has found that not the baseline MAP but its wide fluctuations in the first few days have been related to the 1- and 3-months' poor outcomes [36]. Recently, an observational study has confirmed that the clinical outcome in acute IS depends not only on initial BP levels, but also on the direction and magnitude of BP changes over the first 24–48 h [37].

The mechanisms of the transitory BP elevation and its fluctuations in acute IS are not well understood. Elevated BP in acute IS may present a compensatory response, maintaining an adequate brain perfusion. The available data suggest that the focal cerebral ischemia is the main underlying cause of acute transitory hypertensive response. BP declines when the collateral blood supply has become sufficient and the regional CBF has been restored. The spontaneous reduction of BP after vessel recanalization [20] implies this mechanism. Stress responses to hospitalization and neurological deficits with autonomic nervous system activation and raised plasma catecholamines [15–16] also contribute to BP elevation in acute IS.

Although it has been pointed out that quantitative assessments are required to evaluate the effects of vasoactive drugs on cerebral perfusion in acute IS, no randomized clinical trials have focused on this issue [3]. Recently, a study has shown that testing of the dynamic cerebral autoregulation capacity could be a promising tool to determine the risk of hypoperfision and cerebral ischemia, especially in elderly subjects [38]. Bilateral TDS and continuous arterial BP recording have also been used for assessment of the dynamic cerebral autoregulation in patients with head injury, admitted to the intensive care unit [39]. The employment of bedside TDS has been suggested as a useful method to determine individual safe limits when MAP is lowered in acute IS [27]. However, neither past nor ongoing trials on the effects of antihypertensive treatment in acute IS have included in their protocols monitoring of cerebral hemodynamics. Taking into account the effects of severe carotid artery disease on cerebral perfusion during BP lowering in acute IS, extracranial Doppler should also be performed.

Obviously, ultrasound carotid artery disease assessment and cerebral hemodynamics monitoring, using bilateral TDS, should be performed during the emergency BP management in acute IS, with the aim to maintain adequate perfusion of the penumbral tissue and prevent infarct enlargement   Such an

14

approach could individualize the antihypertensive treatment in acute IS and improve its long-term functional outcome [40].

In addition, several experimental studies have shown that numerous medications limit the cellular effects of acute cerebral ischemia or reperfusion. However, the interventions with the available neuroprotective agents have not found an improvement of the clinical outcome after an acute IS. Moreover in some trials the treated patients had a poorer outcome   in comparison with the controls. This is why these medications are not recommended   for treatment of   acute stroke patients [7, 35]. At present, the thrombolysis and the maintenance of an adequate penumbral perfusion is the most important treatment strategy for patients with acute IS.

An additional consideration requires the ischemic penumbra, initially defined as an ischemic zone with reduced regional CBF and absent electrical activity in which the ion homeostasis is not irreversibly disturbed. Ischemic penumbra is also characterized as a region of insufficient blood supply in which energy metabolism is still preserved. Moreover and in contrast with infarction, in penumbral tissue the glucose metabolic rate is preserved or even enhanced and the metabolic disturbances are reversible if the blood supply is restored or if the brain tissue could be metabolically protected [41]. The ischemic penumbra is associated with acute IS and the restoration of the blood flow to penumbral tissue may facilitate recovery and improve outcome in stroke patients.

Although the etiology and pathogenesis of IS and TIA and their prevention strategies are similar, relatively few studies have been focused on the transient elevated BP in TIA patients. These two clinical manifestations of cerebrovascular diseases are caused by a large artery disease, cardiac emboli and a small artery disease. However, they differ with the severity of the local brain ischemia revealed by multimodal MRI.

In TIA patients, perfusion weighted imaging (PWI) obtained 2 hours after a symptom onset, reveals a hypoperfused area relevant to the neurological deficit, while diffusion-weighted imaging (DWI) is considered normal. However, a follow-up DWI after 3 days shows diffusion abnormalities of the initially hypoperfused area.

Evidently, the hypoperfusion in TIA patients could proceed to a cerebral infarction or reduce to a benign oligemia, which does not cause neurological symptoms. Therefore, from a pathophysiological viewpoint, TIA could be defined as an ischemic penumbra of varied duration with clinical symptoms, usually lasting less than one hour [42].

It could be also pointed out that the TIA is not a benign condition. It has been reported that a preceding TIA occurs in 7% to 40% of the patients with a first IS. For these reasons, an agreement has been reached that TIA patients should be treated as medical emergencies [43].

Few studies have focused on the BP course in patients with TIA. A transient elevated BP after the events has been recorded in 67% of the patients on the day of admission. It decreases spontaneously in the first days after the onset of TIA, mainly on the second day to a plateau level, which has been reached on the fifth day. Only 5% of the patients remain hypertensives until discharge from the hospital. BP falls to normotensive levels in most patients [44].

These findings show that the course of BP after TA and acute IS is similar. The pathophysiology of the transient BP elevation in acute IS and in TIA is also similar. The elevated BP in patients with TIA might be caused by the stress at hospital admission, following by activation of the sympathetic adrenomedullar pathways.

In patients with TIA an elevated plasma catecholamine concentration has been also observed. The high plasma norepinephrine in these patients could give rise to an increase in peripheral sympathetic activity [14]. The focal cerebral hypoperfusion in TIA may also contribute to transient BP elevation.

It has been reported that BP lowering does not reduce the risk of IS in patients with previous TIA. About 20% of patients with TIA or IS have significant stenosis or occlusion of at least 1 carotid artery. However, in the trials of BP lowering after IS or TIA they have not been recorded [32].

It should be mentioned that well designed clinical trials on the antihypertensive treatment in patients with TIA and evidence-based guidelines are not yet available. Evidently, a panel consensus on this issue is needed.

The available data show that the BP lowering in patients with acute IS may compromise the blood supply of the ischemic penumbra and cause infarct enlargement. In TIA patients the aggressive BP lowering may also not be safe, because the ischemic penumbra could proceed to cerebral infarction. That is why a routine BP lowering in acute IS and TIA should not be recommended.

The dilemma not to treat or to treat elevated BP in acute IS could be resolved by appropriate BP management. The antihypertensive treatment should depend on clinical characteristics, ultrasound carotid artery disease assessment and on cerebral hemodynamics, evaluated by bedside bilateral transcranial ultrasonography. The cerebral hemodynamics monitoring may contribute to maintaining of an adequate penumbral perfusion and prevent infarct enlargement. Such an approach could individualize the antihypertensive treatment in acute IS and to result in better clinical outcomes.

Conclusion

An elevated BP is a frequent finding in patients with acute IS and in the next few days, it declines spontaneously. The mechanisms of the transient BP elevation are not fully understood. Data are available that the mental stress and cerebral ischemia are the main underlying causes and the recanalization could contribute to the BP decline.

Probably, the elevated systemic BP in acute IS may have beneficial effect in maintaining an adequate cerebral perfusion pressure. The BP lowering in acute IS could lead to infarct enlargement and poor outcomes. There are increasing evidence that the antihypertensive treatment may be not required in the first few hours of acute IS onset.

The present guidelines for BP management in acute IS are not evidence-based. Clinical trials have reported that BP lowering in acute IS may be associated with a poor functional outcome, probably because of impaired CBF autoregulation and failure of collateral blood supply. The severe carotid artery stenosis or occlusion may compromise the cerebral blood supply when the systematic BP falls. The carotid

18

disease is a frequent finding in IS and TIA and has an important role in their pathogenesis. However, the presence or severity of carotid disease have been recorded only in one randomized controlled trial on antihypertensive treatment in acute IS.

The carotid artery stenosis severity assessment and cerebral hemodynamics monitoring in the course of antihypertensive treatment in acute IS should be performed with the aim to maintain an adequate cerebral perfusion. The ultrasound carotid artery stenosis evaluation and monitoring of cerebral hemodinamics, using bilateral TDS, could be useful tools to guide and individualize the BP management in acute IS aimed at prevention of infarct enlargement and better functional outcomes. Prospective studies are needed to confirm such a treatment strategy.

At present, although the experimental studies have shown that numerous medications reduce the ischemic cerebral lesions, clinical trials have not found a beneficial effects from neuroprotective agents in patients with IS and they are not recommended for these patients. New neuroprotective medications and well designed clinical studies should clarify the role of neuroprotection in acute stroke.

References

1. Wallace JD, Levy LL. Blood pressure after stroke. JAMA 1981; 246:2177–80.
2. Britton M, Carlsson A, de Faire U. Blood pressure course in patients with acute stroke and matched controls. Stroke 1986; 17:861–4.
3. Bath P, Boysen G, Donnan G, et al. Hypertension in acute stroke: what to do? Stroke 2001; 32:1697–98.

4. Leonardi-Bee J, Bath PM, Phillips SJ, Sandercock PA; IST Collaborative Group. Blood pressure and clinical outcomes in the International Stroke Trial. Stroke 2002; 33:1315–20.

5. Qureshi AI, Ezzeddine MA, Nasar A, et al. Prevalence of elevated blood pressure in 563,704 adult patients with stroke presenting to the ED in the United States. Am J Emerg Med 2007; 25:32–8.

6. Qureshi AI. Acute hypertensive response in patients with stroke: pathophysiology and management. Circulation 2008; 118:176–87.

7. Adams HP Jr, del Zoppo G, Alberts MJ, et al. Guidelines for the early management of adults with ischemic stroke: a guideline from the American Heart Association/American Stroke Association Stroke Council, Clinical Cardiology Council, Cardiovascular Radiology and Intervention Council, and the Atherosclerotic Peripheral Vascular Disease and Quality of Care Outcomes in Research Interdisciplinary Working Groups: the American Academy of Neurology affirms the value of this guideline as an educational tool for neurologists. Stroke 2007; 38:1655–711.

8. Aiyagari V, Gorelick PB. Management of blood pressure for acute and recurrent stroke. Stroke 2009; 40:2251–56.

9. Horn J, Limburg M. Calcium antagonists for ischemic stroke: a systematic review. Stroke 2001; 32:570–6.

10. Geeganage C, Bath PM. Vasoactive drugs for acute stroke. Cochrane Database Syst Rev 2010; 7: CD002839.

11. Sandset EC, Bath PM, Boysen G, et al.; SCAST Study Group. The angiotensinreceptor blocker candesartan for treatment of acute stroke (SCAST): a randomised, placebo-controlled, double-blind trial. Lancet 2011; 377:741–50.

12. Lisk DR, Grotta JC, Lamki LM, et al. Should hypertension be treated after acute stroke? A randomized controlled trial using single photon emission computed tomography. Arch Neurol 1993; 50:855–62.

13. Carlberg B, Asplund K, Hagg E. Factors influencing admission blood pressure levels in patients with acute stroke. Stroke 1991; 22:527–30.

14. Myers MG, Norris JW, Hachniski VC, Sole MJ. Plasma norepinephrine in stroke. Stroke 1981; 12:200–4.

15. Olsson T, Astrom M, Eriksson S, Forssell A. Hypercortisolism revealed by the dexamethasone suppression test in patients [corrected] with acute ischemic stroke. Stroke 1989; 20:1685–90.

16. Olsson T, Marklund N, Gustafson Y, Nasman B. Abnormalities at different levels of the hypothalamic-pituitary-adrenocortical axis early after stroke. Stroke 1992;23:1573–6.

17. Chamorro A, Amaro S, Vargas M, et al. Catecholamines, infection, and death in acute ischemic stroke. J Neurol Sci 2007; 252:29–35.

18. Ito A, Omae T, Katsuki S. Acute changes in blood pressure following vascular diseases in the brain stem. Stroke 1973; 4:80–4.

19. Hilz MJ, Devinsky O, Szczepanska H, Borod JC, Marthol H, Tutaj M. Right ventromedial prefrontal lesions result in paradoxical cardiovascular activation with emotional stimuli. Brain 2006; 129:3343–55.

20. Mattle HP, Kappeler L, Arnold M, et al. Blood pressure and vessel recanalization in the first hours after ischemic stroke. Stroke 2005; 36:264–8.

21. Yatsu FM, Zivin J. Hypertension in acute ischemic strokes. Not to treat. Arch Neurol 1985; 42:999–1000.

22. Spence JD, Del Maestro RF. Hypertension in acute ischemic strokes. Treat. Arch Neurol 1985; 42:1000–2.

23. Ahmed N, Nasman P, Wahlgren NG. Effect of intravenous nimodipine on blood pressure and outcome after acute stroke. Stroke 2000; 31:1250–5.

24. Castillo J, Leira R, Garcia MM, Serena J, Blanco M, Davalos A. Blood pressure decrease during the acute phase of ischemic stroke is associated with brain injury and poor stroke outcome. Stroke 2004; 35:520–6.

25. Hanson SK, Grotta JC, Rhoades H, et al. Value of single-photon emission-computed tomography in acute stroke therapeutic trials. Stroke 1993; 24:1322–9.

26. Dawson SL, Panerai RB, Potter JF. Serial changes in static and dynamic cerebral autoregulation after acute ischaemic stroke. Cerebrovasc Dis 2003; 16:69–75.

27. Powers WJ, Videen TO, Diringer MN, Aiyagari V, Zazulia AR. Autoregulation after ischaemic stroke. J Hypertens 2009; 27:2218–22.

28. Sare GM, Gray LJ, Bath PM. Effect of antihypertensive agents on cerebral blood flow and flow velocity in acute ischaemic stroke: systematic review of controlled studies. J Hypertens 2008; 26:1058–64.

29. van der Grond J, Balm R, Kappelle LJ, Eikelboom BC, Mali WP. Cerebral metabolism of patients with stenosis or occlusion of the internal carotid artery. A 1H-MR spectroscopic imaging study. Stroke 1995; 26:822–8.

30. Grubb RL Jr, Derdeyn CP, Fritsch SM, et al. Importance of hemodynamic factors in the prognosis of symptomatic carotid occlusion. JAMA 1998;280:1055–60.

31. Vernieri F, Pasqualetti P, Passarelli F, Rossini PM, Silvestrini M. Outcome of carotid artery occlusion is predicted by cerebrovascular reactivity. Stroke 1999;30:593–8.

32. Rothwell PM, Howard SC, Spence JD; Carotid Endarterectomy Trialists'Collaboration. Relationship between blood pressure and stroke

risk in patients with symptomatic carotid occlusive disease. Stroke 2003; 34:2583–90.

33. Sare GM, Gray LJ, Wardlaw J, Chen C, Bath PM; ENOS Trial Investigators. Is lowering blood pressure hazardous in patients with significant ipsilateral carotid stenosis and acute ischaemic stroke? Interim assessment in the 'Efficacy of Nitric Oxide in Stroke' trial. Blood Press Monit 2009; 14:20–5.

34. Strandgaard S. Autoregulation of cerebral circulation in hypertension. Acta Neurol Scand Suppl 1978;66:1–82.

35. European Stroke Organisation (ESO) Executive Committee; ESO Writing Committee. Guidelines for management of ischaemic stroke and transient ischaemic attack 2008. Cerebrovasc Dis 2008; 25:457–507.

36. Aslanyan S, Fazekas F, Weir CJ, Horner S, Lees KR; GAIN International Steering Committee and Investigators. Effect of blood pressure during the acute period of ischemic stroke on stroke outcome: a tertiary analysis of the GAIN International Trial. Stroke 2003; 34:2420–5.

37. Ntaios G, Lambrou D, Michel P. Blood pressure change and outcome in acute ischemic stroke: the impact of baseline values, previous hypertensive disease and previous antihypertensive treatment. J Hypertens 2011; 29:1583–9.

38. van Beek AH, Claassen JA, Rikkert MG, Jansen RW. Cerebral autoregulation: an overview of current concepts and methodology with special focus on the elderly. J Cereb Blood Flow Metab 2008;28:1071–85.

39. Aaslid R, Blaha M, Sviri G, Douville CM, Newell DW. Asymmetric dynamic cerebral autoregulatory response to cyclic stimuli. Stroke 2007; 38:1465-9.

40. Hadjiev DI, Mineva PP. Elevated blood pressure management in acute ischemic stroke remains controversial: could this issue be resolved? Med Hypotheses. 2013; 80(1):50-2.

41. Ginsberg MD. Injury mechanisms in the ischemic penumbra – approaches to acute ischemic stroke. Cerebrovasc Dis 1997; 7 (Suppl 2): 7–12.

42. Hadjiev DI, Mineva PP A reappraisal of the definition and pathophysiology of the transient ischemic attack. Med Sci Monit. 2007 Mar;13(3):50-53.

43. Sacco RL: Risk factors for TIA and TIA as a risk factor for stroke. Neurology, 2004; 62, Suppl 6: S7–S11

44. Jansen PA, Schulte BP, Poels EF, Gribnau FW. Course of blood pressure after cerebral infarction and transient ischemic attack. Clin Neurol Neurosurg. 1987; 89(4):243–6.

Chapter 2.

Blood Pressure Management and Cognitive Functions in Elderly Hypertensive Patients

Introduction

Hypertension is the most important modifiable risk factor for vascular cognitive impairment (VCI) and vascular dementia (VaD) in elderly hypertensive persons without a history of stroke [1-5].

There is strong evidence that older hypertensive patients benefit from antihypertensive therapy in terms of reduced cardiovascular morbidity and mortality [6,7]. However, the impact of antihypertensive treatment on the incidence of VCI and VaD in elderly hypertensive patients without a history of stroke is still a matter of debate. Moreover, the targets of BP lowering in elderly hypertensive persons are not yet determined. Data emerge that BP lowering beyond a certain level in elderly persons could increase the risk of cerebral hypoperfusion and cognitive decline [8]. However, in elderly hypertensive patients, the cerebral hemodynamics has not been monitored in the course of antihypertensive treatment.

In addition, the targets of BP lowering may depend on different medical conditions such as extracranial occlusive disease, cardiac disease, diabetes mellitus (DM) and renal impairment [9].

Besides, the pathogenesis of VCI is not completely solved. Obviously, with the increasing age-related risk of hypertension [10] and the consequent vascular cognitive disorders, antihypertensive therapy in elderly hypertensive patients will attain great medical importance with a huge public health economic burden. Probably, an appropriate BP management in elderly hypertensive patients may prevent or slow dawn cognitive decline.

Epidemiology of the vascular cognitive impairment in hypertension
Several cross-sectional and longitudinal population epidemiological studies, using different designs and patient populations, have focused on the relationships between hypertension and cognitive disorders.

Cross-sectional population epidemiological studies. In a review of 16 cross-sectional studies, including 19,501 subjects, the evidence from completed randomized controlled trials of BP reduction on cognitive performance have been analyzed. Conflicting relationships between BP reduction and cognitive performance have been found. The data have shown that BP lowering may have a heterogeneous effect on different aspects of cognitive function [11].

Another cross-sectional study has shown that persons with very advanced age, 75-101 years, and SBP below 130 mmHg tend to be at high risk of cognitive impairment, assessed by the Mini Mental State Examination (MMSE), while those with SBP of 160-179 mmHg have a lower risk of cognitive decline. These results suggest that SBP of at least 130 mmHg is important to the maintenance of cognitive functioning in the very old persons. However, the subjects with severe, poorly controlled hypertension are at risk of worsening of the cognitive performance (12). In the oldest patients, an association between lower SBP and the risk of cognitive impairment has been also reported. The cognitive functions have been evaluated by the MMSE (13).

Longitudinal population epidemiological studies. The impact of elevated midlife SBP on cognitive function has been demonstrated by several longitudinal epidemiological studies. It has been reported that midlife hypertension in men is associated with cognitive impairment and dementia later in life. The risk of cognitive dysfunctions increases progressively with the increasing level of midlife SBP. However, the level of cognitive function is not associated with midlife DBP. There is also evidence that the risk of dementia, including Alzheimer's disease, increases among older adults with untreated or poorly controlled hypertension. It is pointed out that the early control of SBP may reduce the risk of cognitive impairment in old age [14-16].

A longitudinal epidemiological study has analyzed the individual changes in SBP over a 30-year interval and their association with neuropsychological outcome in old age. A relatively small group of persons have maintained elevated SBP over the life span, despite the use of antihypertensive drugs. These persons have been at increased risk for reduced verbal learning and memory functions. On the other hand, the persons who have experienced a decreased SPB have been at risk for decreased psychomotor speed [17].

Furthermore, it has been shown that patients with high midlife SBP experience cognitive dysfunctions as well as brain atrophy and increased volume of white matter hyperintensities on MRI in late life. It is suggested that the long-term impact of elevated SBP on decline in late-life neurobehavioral functioning is mediated through its chronic negative effect on brain tissue [18]. A longitudinal population study of healthy elderly men, lasting 20 years, found that the high DBP at baseline has predicted an impairment of the cognitive functions later in life]19]. Another longitudinal population-based study has indicated that higher levels of baseline SBP, DBP and mean arterial pressure have been significantly associated with cognitive decline [20].

A comprehensive longitudinal study has analyzed the relation between BP and development of dementia in age intervals 70-75, 75-79 and 79-85 years in subjects non-demented at age 70. The sample has been followed up for 15 years. It has been found that the participants with WMLs on computed tomography at age 85 have higher BP at age 70 than those without such lesions. In the years before dementia onset BP decreases to the levels similar to or lower than in non-demented subjects. It is concluded that previously higher BP may increase the risk of dementia by inducing small-vessel disease and WMLs. However, it remains unclear to what extend the BP decline before dementia onset is a consequence or a cause of the brain lesions [14].

On the other hand several longitudinal epidemiological studies have not found a relationship between hypertension and cognitive disorders in elderly persons. In a biracial longitudinal population study among persons aged 65 or more, no association was found between high BP at the beginning of the observation and cognitive decline after a 6-year follow-up period [21]. Furthermore, in elderly persons on antihypertensive therapy, an inverse association between BP levels and dementia has been reported. The risk of dementia decreases with increasing BP levels [22].

In a population case-control study of elderly hypertensive patients, only negative correlation between DBP and cognitive performance has been reported Another study found that hypertension is not a risk factor for age-related memory disorders [23].

Despite the inconsistent findings concerning the association of hypertension with cognitive functions, it seems that high midlife BP enhances the cognitive decline in late life but in old age, mild hypertension may improve the cognitive performance. These data suggest that early and adequate treatment of the high midlife BP could decrease the risk of cognitive impairment in late life. However, aggressive BP lowering in elderly hypertensive patients may be harmful.

The largest long-term longitudinal epidemiological studies providing evidence for an association between elevated BP and cognitive decline in the elderly subjects are shown in Table 1.

However, hypertension is often accompanied by other vascular risk factors (VRF) such as dyslipidemias, cardiac diseases, particularly atrial fibrillation, DM and carotid intimal-medial thickness, which may also contribute to the development of VCI and VaD. The role of the additional VRF has not been considered in the most of longitudinal population epidemiological studies on the association of hypertension with cognitive disorders.

Table 1. Longitudinal population epidemiological studies on the association between blood pressure and cognitive function

Authors	Sample size at entry	Age at entry (years)	Follow-up (years)	Conclusion
Launer et al. [15]	3735 men	52.7± 4.7	25	High SBP in midlife is associated with cognitive dysfunction in late life
Swan et al. [18]	717	39 to 59	30	High SBP is associated with reduced verbal learning and memory
Kilander et al. [19]	999 men	50	20	High DBP predicts a cognitive impairment in late life
Elias et al. [20]	529	47 to 83	20	Higher SBP, and DBP are associated with cognitive decline

Pathogenesis of the vascular cognitive impairment in hypertension

According to the newer research classification systems VCI has been defined as a syndrome taking into account the spectrum of cognitive domains, at least one, which often includes executive dysfunction and the various types of brain vascular diseases that could underlie cognitive symptoms. The focal cerebral ischemia and subclinical vascular brain damages are also included. The most severe form of VCI is VaD. It is pointed out that new studies are needed to further our understanding of VCI and to better characterize its neuropsychological profile. Studies of intensive reduction of VRF in high-risk patients are also an important research priority [24].

Several studies are focused on cerebral hemodynamics and on cerebral structural changes, evaluated by neuroimaging in hypertensive patients with the aim to clarify the pathogenesis of the cognitive impairment in hypertension. However, because the PWI is not widely available, the cerebral perfusion abnormalities in hypertensive patients with VCI without a history of stroke or TIA are not frequently recorded.

The first study on the CBF and metabolism in patients with uncomplicated essential hypertension was performed more than 60 years ago using the nitrous oxide method. It found a marked and consistent increase in cerebrovascular resistance, while the global CBF and cerebral oxygen consumption remained in normal limits. It suggested that in hypertension, there may be a primary cerebrovascular constriction, accompanied by a compensatory hypertension, which maintains a normal CBF. The marked increase in cerebrovascular resistance could be explained by development of functional and structural changes in the cerebral small vessels caused by hypertension.

In patients with chronic hypertension, the increased cerebrovascular resistance causes a change in the CBF autoregulation. The lower and the upper autoregulation limits are shifted to higher pressure levels owing to structural changes in the cerebral small vessels. This vascular adaptation protects the brain against high intravascular pressure but makes it more vulnerable to ischemia at low BP. In some patients the antihypertensive therapy does not influence the low limit of CBF autoregulation [25]. Thus, excessive BP lowering may compromise the brain blood supply to such an extent that neurological dysfunctions or death occur. An understanding of the problem requires detailed knowledge of the pathophysiology of the cerebral circulation in hypertension [26,27].

Studies on the regional CBF (rCBF), measured by the 33Xe inhalation method, in neurologically asymptomatic hypertensive patients have shown reductions in blood flow more marked in the frontal, temporal and parietal regions. Regional temporal lobe impairment has been also noted in the newly diagnosed and treated subjects. A significant correlation has been found between rCBF and mean arterial BP. It is pointed out that rCBF examination presents a relatively simple technique to explore the cerebral perfusion in hypertensive persons [26–30].

In older hypertensive persons using repeated positron-emission tomography longitudinal rCBF, changes assessed over a period of 6 years have been found that differ from healthy controls. In hypertensive patients, rCBF decreases have been observed in prefrontal, anterior cingulate, occipital areas and hippocampus in comparison with controls. However, relevant cognitive impairment have not been demonstrated The results have shown that hypertension significantly affects resting brain function in older persons and the duration of hypertension contributes to the patterns of changes over time [31]. The patterns of longitudinal rCBF changes without apparent cognitive dysfunctions could be considered a subclinical stage of cognitive impairment.

Functional neuroimaging studies, using positron emission tomography (PET), in hypertensive patients have also found a reduction in regional cerebral metabolic rates for glucose in some subcortical nuclei and in the border zone between anterior and middle cerebral arteries which is vulnerable to ischemia from carotid disease, systemic hypotension or both. These hypertensive patients may have experienced ischemia severe enough to cause border zone reduction of functional neuronal connectivity as a result of carotid pathology, antihypertensive treatment or hypotensive episodes with a right-shifted autoregulation curve [32,33].

The cerebral hemodynamics in asymptomatic hypertensive patients has been studied by TDS. An association between a low CBF, measured with transcranial Doppler, and cognitive impairments in patients aged 55 years or older has been reported. A relationship between silent WMLs on magnetic resonance imaging (MRI) and impaired cerebral autoregulation has been shown. Blood flow velocities have been found to correlate positively with SBP, but they have been negatively related to the duration of hypertension [34, 35].

Silent cerebral infarctions in the brain areas supplied by perforating arterioles on MRI are frequent findings in older hypertensive patients. These data suggest that hypertensive arterioles changes play a crucial rope in the occurrence of silent cerebral infarction [36]. High prevalence of WMLs and ventricular enlargement on MRI has been found among elderly hypertensive subjects. The MRI abnormalities have been accompanied by cognitive dysfunctions. The hypertensive patients have tended to perform worse when they have been assessed for attention and visiopractical skills [37].

In patients with essential hypertension, without a history of stroke, quantitative volumetric MRI has shown atrophies in the thalamic nuclei and temporal lobes, attended with poor memory performance. This study has also found that hypertension exacerbates the brain atrophies due to advanced age. The strongest interaction of age and hypertension has been observed in the temporal and occipital lobes [38]. In elderly people, including subjects with mild hypertension, the subcortical gray and white matter hyperintensities on MRI have been found to correlate with the impairments of attention and executive functions [39].

WMLs on MRI and lacunes, most consistently associated with hypertension and DM, are the essential lesions in patients with VCI without a history of stroke. DBP seems to be an important risk factor related to the progression of these lesions. It has been found that both high and declining DBP are associated with cortical atrophy and more severe periventricular WMLs on MRI [40,41]. Older hypertensive patients have had smaller whole brain volumes and increased burden of periventricular and subcortical, frontal and temporal, WMLs [42].

In addition several longitudinal studies have focused on the association of low BP in elderly persons with the risk of cognitive impairment. The low DBP has been reported to increase the risk of dementia in elderly subjects over 75 years of age [43], probably by affecting a cerebral perfusion [44]. A marked decrease in BP over 3 years before dementia diagnosis and afterward has also been found. A greater decline in SBP is associated with increased risk of dementia only in older people with low BP or affected by vascular disorders [45]. A longitudinal observational population-based study has reported that the lower SBP in individuals 80 years and older is associated with an increased risk of cognitive impairment [46].

The available data show that functional and later structural changes of the cerebral small vessels, supplying the deep and periventricular white matter and basal ganglia, play a crucial role in the development of subcortical ischemic damage, leading to a VCI, which is characterized by a specific cognitive profile, involving preserved memory with impairments of attention and executive function [47, 48]. Obviously, hypoperfusion and ischemia in these regions occur as a result of both an increase in cerebrovascular resistance and a decrease in CBF by excessive BP lowering. Age and long-standing hypertension are the most important causes for these lesions.

Besides, hypertension is frequently accompanied by other vascular risk factors (VRF) [49–51]. The additional vascular risk factors, particularly DM, accompanying hypertension may contribute to the development of subcortical ischemic lesions and VCI. Some studies have shown that the cerebral WMLs are frequently related to DM. It has been established that age and DM are independent predictors of cerebral WMLs [52]. Hypertension is also associated with carotid atherosclerosis [53]. It has been shown that the SBP is independently related to carotid atherosclerosis, assessed by ultrasonography [54, 55]. Although the role of the asymptomatic carotid stenosis in the development of cognitive impairment is not yet clear [56], there is evidence that the asymptomatic high-grade stenosis of the left internal carotid artery is an independent risk factor for cognitive impairment and decline [57]. It has also been reported that subjects with asymptomatic carotid stenosis have poorer neuropsychological performance, independent of the cerebral WMLs [58].

The well- and less well-documented modifiable VRF often occur in clusters. Vascular risk factors are also known to interact and to multiply the risk of stroke and VCI.

Different combinations of risk factors for stroke and VCI have been described. The Framingham profile consisting of elevated SBP, dyslipidemia, glucose intolerance, cigarette smoking and left ventricular hypertrophy identifies persons at highest risk of stroke. The clusters of three or more than three risk factors accompanying hypertension occur at four times the rate expected by chance [49]. It has been shown that multiple, two or more, risk factors are more prevalent in hypertensive patients (55.5%) than in no-hypertensive controls (6.5%). Obesity, followed by dyslipidemia, current cigarette smoking and DM are the most frequent risk factors accompanying hypertension [59].

The findings from the Northern Manhattan Study have shown that the metabolic syndrome, which includes hypertension, diabetes mellitus, obesity, low HDL-cholesterol levels and high triglycerides is a highly prevalent constellation of multiple risk factors. It has also been reported that the metabolic syndrome is significantly associated with IS, especially in women [60].

A population-based longitudinal epidemiological study has focused on the prevalence and the distribution patterns of multiple vascular risk factors for IS. Three or more modifiable risk factors have been detected in 52% of the subjects without a history of stroke. Dyslipidemias, hypertension, obesity, current cigarette smoking and cardiac diseases have been found to be the most prevalent individual risk factors among the subjects with multiple modifiable VRF. After a 2-year follow-up 2.7% of the persons with multiple VRF have reached the end points: TIA, IS and myocardial infarction. Hypertension, cardiac diseases, high LDL-cholesterol levels, obesity have been found the most prevalent VRF among persons with multiple risk factors, who reached an outcome end point. It is suggested that as far as multiple risk factors could cause pronounced chronic cerebral hypoperfusion a benefit may be provided by neuroprotection. The identification of persons with multiple VRF would allow their selection for primary multimodal stroke prevention [51].

The population–based epidemiological studies show considerable geographic and race-ethnic differences in the prevalence and in the distribution patterns of multiple risk factors for IS and VCI. Evidently, the presence of the metabolic syndrome identifies patients at increased risk of TIA, IS and VCI.

The available data suggest that cerebral WMLs, a consequence of small vessel disease, and probably the high-grade carotid stenosis, contribute to the development of cognitive disorders in elderly hypertensive patients. The main risk factors for these lesions are age, hypertension and DM. Besides, certain observational studies showed that low BP in elderly persons increases the risk of cognitive impairment [61, 62].

It has been pointed out that the progression of leukoaraiosis, a frequent finding in elderly hypertensive patients, accelerates the cognitive decline. The worsening of cognitive functions has been found 4 times faster in patients with the greatest progression of leukoaraiosis, The cognitive correlates of leukoaraiosis correspond to the subcorical pattern of impaired frontal and executive functions [61].

Furthermore, it seems that the cerebral WMLs and lacunar infarction may be associated with some genetic factors, particularly a polymorphism of the angiotensin-converting enzyme gene. A significant interaction between hypertension, apoE ε 4 allele and subcortical, but not periventricular, WMLs has been reported (72). Probably, the genetic risk factors for deep subcortical and periventricular WMLs are not the same. However, it is pointed out that the lack of a clear determination of the phenotype is an important factor limiting the study of genetic factors of VCI, because superimposed Alzheimer disease processes cannot be ruled out [24].

While the epidemiological studies are mainly focused on the relationship between individual VRF and cognitive functions, the studies on the relationship between multiple vascular risk factors in elderly patients without a history of stroke and cognition are scanty.

In a cross-sectional study, including nondemented elderly persons, the relationship between well-documented VRF and cognitive functions has been assessed. The persons with 3 or more VRF have shown significantly more impaired executive functions and speed of information processing than the persons without any risk factors. Hypertension, absence of physical activity and smoking have been found the most frequent VRF. Hypertension has been reported in 79% of the persons with 3 or more VRF and in 40 % in those with 1 or 2 VRF. It is pointed out that the prevention and early treatment of hypertension as well as lifestyle modifications might contribute to maintain a better level of cognitive functioning [63]

Obviously, new well designed studies are needed to evaluate the impact of different combinations of VRFs on the cognitive functions in elderly hypertensive patients without a history of stroke.

Antihypertensive treatment in elderly hypertensive patients and cognition

Five randomized, placebo-controlled trials have focused on the efficacy of antihypertensive treatment in preventing cognitive disorders in elderly hypertensive patients without a history of stroke.

The Systolic Hypertension in Elderly Program (SHEP) study has shown no significant difference in the cognitive performance, evaluated by neuropsychological tests, between patients receiving antihypertensive treatment – diuretic (chlorthalidone), and/or beta-blocker (atenolol) or reserpine, and a control group [64].

The Medical Research Council (MRC) trial, a randomized, placebo-controlled, single blind trial of hypertension in older adults includes 2584 persons, 65–74 years of age. The participants have had mean SBP of 160–209 mmHg and mean DBP< 115 mmHg. The cognitive functions have been evaluated by the Paired Associative Learning Test (PALT) and the Trial Making Test (TMT). The study has not found any difference in the cognitive functions between subjects on antihypertensive drugs – diuretic (hydrochlorthiazide) and/or beta-blocker (atenolol), and a placebo group [65].

In the Systolic Hypertension in Europe (Syst-Eur) trial, a significant reduction by 50% of the incidence of dementia has been reported among patients with isolated systolic hypertension, receiving dihydropyridine calcium channel blocker (nitrendipine) with or without angiotensin-converting enzyme inhibitor (enalapril) and/or diuretic (hydrochlorthiazide). Cognitive functions have been assessed by the MMSE and the diagnosis of dementia has been based on the criteria of the Diagnostic and Statistical Manual of Mental Disorders, third edition, revised. A slight improvement in MMSE scores with decreasing DBP has been observed. It has been suggested that the beneficial effect could be partly explain by neuroprotective properties of the dihydropyridine calcium channel blocker [66].

The Study on Cognition and Prognosis in the Elderly (SCOPE) is one of the largest prevention studies on cognitive impairment and dementia in patients with mild hypertension, SBP 160–179 mmHg and/or DBP 90–99 mmHg. No differences in the cognitive decline, evaluated by MMSE, have been found between the patients receiving angiotensin II receptor blocker (candesartan) and the control group [67]. A positive effect has only been seen in elderly persons with slightly low cognitive function at baseline [68]. However, in this study antihypertensive drugs have been added as needed to control BP in both groups.

The Hypertension in the Very Elderly Trial, cognitive function assessment (HYVET-COG), a double-blind, placebo-controlled trial, has been completed. The study includes 3336 hypertensive elderly patients 80 years of age or older receiving antihypertensive treatment – diuretic (indapamide) and angiotensin-converting enzyme inhibitor (perindopril), added if necessary to achieve the target BP of 150/80 mm Hg, or placebo. The cognitive functions have been assessed at baseline and annually by MMSE. No significant difference in the cognitive decline between treatment and placebo groups has been observed. It is concluded, that the antihypertensive treatment in elderly patients does not statistically reduce incidence of dementia [69].

The randomized placebo-controlled trials assessing the effects of antihypertensive treatment on cognitive performance in elderly hypertensive patients are presented in Table 2.

Several population cohort studies on the efficacy of long-term treatment of hypertension in reducing the risk of cognitive dysfunction have also shown controversial results [62]. A cohort study concluded that in hypertensive men, the duration of the antihypertensive medication longer than 12 years is associated with a significant reduction in the risk of dementia and cognitive decline. In contrast, another longitudinal cohort study in older persons did not find a relationship between BP and risk of Alzheimer's disease or cognitive decline.

Table 2 Randomized controlled trials assessing the effects of antihypertensive treatment on cognitive function

Trials	Sample size	Age (years)	Mean Follow-up (years)	Conclusion
SHEP [64]	2034	≥60	5	No positive effect
MRC [65]	2584	65–74	4.5	No positive effect
Syst-Eur [66]	2418	≥60	2	Risk reduction by 50%
SCOPE [67]	4964	70–89	3.7	No positive effect
HYVET-COG [69]	3336	>80	2.2	No positive effect

Furthermore, in a recent meta-analysis, no convincing evidence has been found that antihypertensive treatment decreases the risk of cognitive disorders in patients with cardiovascular and cerebrovascular diseases or in hypertensive subjects without apparent prior cerebrovascular disease [70]. However, the impact on cognition in these trials has not been considered a primary outcome. Ultrasonography of the carotid arteries and an assessment of the cerebral hemodynamics have not been performed either.

In several population cohort studies controversial effects of antihypertensive treatment in reducing the risk of cognitive impairment have been also reported. The duration of the antihypertensive treatment has been associated with a significant reduction in the risk of cognitive decline and dementia. Another population cohort study has shown that among the antihypertensive drugs used, calcium antagonists only are associated with a decrease in the risk of cognitive decline. In addition, a cross-sectional and longitudinal study has revealed nonlinear relations of BP with cognitive functions. The cognitive decline has been apparent among older individuals with higher SBP. The cross-sectional findings have shown moderate U- and J- shaped relations between BP and cognitive functions. Both high and low BP has been associated with poorer cognitive performance [71]

The controversial results from the previous clinical trials could be attributed to the different patient populations, a wide range of BP levels at entry, varied types of antihypertensive drugs used, and different neuropsychological tests applied to evaluate cognitive performance. Neuroimaging has not been performed and the diagnoses, particularly the cerebral small vessel disease, remain uncertain. The treatment of the associated risk factors, including lifestyle changes, has not been mentioned. Therefore, the studies completed until now do not contribute to answering the question whether antihypertensive treatment, even when long-term, lowers the rate of dementia and cognitive decline in hypertensive subjects without a history of cerebrovascular disease [72]. It is pointed out that the controversial results suggest the need for well-designed clinical trials to determine whether BP lowering is an important intervention for the prevention of cognitive decline in subjects with or   without cerebrovascular disease [61]

It could be concluded that the antihypertensive treatment in elderly subjects does not decrease the risk of cognitive disorders. Evidently, other risk factors accompanied hypertension may play a role in development of cognitive dysfunctions. Furthermore, BP lowering could compromise the cerebral blood supply with consequent worsening of the cognitive functions. In elderly hypertensive patients an assessment of the carotid disease severity is needed and cerebral hemodynamics should be followed-up in the course of antihypertensive treatment.

Neuroprotection in hypertension
The increased risk of WMLs in hypertensive patients is an indication for early neuroprotecion, before the occurrence of ischemic brain lesions presenting with vascular cognitive disorders.

There is evidence that the ACE inhibitors may attenuate remodelling of cerebral arterioles and improve cerebral autoregulation [73–75]. The ACE inhibitors and the angiotensin II receptor blockers (ARBs), via renin-angiotensin blockade may exert vasoprotection and neuroprotection. It is believed that the neuroprotective properties of the ARBs are mediated by increasing the angiotensin II levels and stimulation of AT2 receptors [76–78]. In addition, ACE inhibitors and ARBs have been shown to possess anti-inflammatory actions [79]. These drugs may also have favorable effects on the patient's quality of life and seem to be effective in maintaining cognitive function trough mechanisms other than blood pressure control [80].

Dihydropyridine calcium channel blockers (CCBs) are also thought to possess neuroprotective action and to slow down the cognitive decline in hypertensive subjects. The neuroprotective and anti-atherosclerotic properties of CCBs could be useful in preventing carotid artery disease. Dihydropyridinic derivates may be also of benefit in a cerebral small vessel disease, which leads to lacunar infarct and subcortical VCI and VaD [66,81]. This class of drugs has been shown to attenuate the progression of atherosclerosis due to its anti-inflammatory and antioxidant actions. In addition, a meta-analysis of 28 trials showed that CCBs are superior to ACE inhibitors for stroke prevention. The prevention from stroke by these drugs has been found to be unrelated to the degree of SBP reduction [82]. It has also been reported that calcium antagonists decrease the risk of cognitive impairment and Alzheimer's disease in elderly hypertensive patients, suggesting a specific neuroprotective effect of these drugs [83].

It has been supposed that statins may exert cholesterol-independent neuroprotective effect in cerebral ischemia that likely attenuates its influence on the brain vasculature and parenchyma. The mechanisms of statins neuroprotection are complex. Several animal studies have shown that statins reduce brain infarct size and improves the neurological outcome by directly up-regulating the brain endothelial nitric oxide synthase (eNOS) and endogenous tissue plasminogen activator (tPA). In addition, they suppress the inflammatory cytokine response both in the vasculature and in the nervous system, especially in the ischemic penumbra, and possess antioxidant activity, which may also contribute to neuroprotection. Emerging data suggest that statins may slow down the cognitive decline and dementia. Probably, if potential cholesterol-independent effects of statins proved to be clinically important, these drugs will be of benefit in the management of a variety of cerebrovascular entities in patients with and without hypercholesterolemia.

Additionally, statins reduce the incidence of IS through beneficial effects on the carotid atherosclerosis [84,85]. Statins have been also found to attenuate the NMDA-induced excitotoxic neuronal death and exhibit direct neuroprotection. They have the potential to render cortical neurons more resistant to NMDA-induced excitotoxic death as a result of changes in cell cholesterol homeostasis [86,87].

The potential neuroprotective properties of statins are presented in Table 3.

It has been reported that the prestroke use of antiplatelet drugs in combination with ACE inhibitors and statins may reduce the stroke severity and the volume of the ischemic tissue at risk, assessed by perfusion-weighted imaging-diffusion-weighted imaging mismatch [88].

Table 3. Neuroprotective properties of statins

- Increase the eNOS activity

    * Increase the cerebral blood flow

    * Decrease infarct size in animals

- Anti-inflammatory effects

- Reduce the oxidative stress

- Increase the tPA activity

- Modulate the NMDA-receptors, inhibit the glutamate

    excitotoxicity and increase the intracellular K

Clinical studies have shown advantages of the combination of both CCBs and statins. An addition of CCBs to statins acts synergistically in retarding the progression of atherosclerosis. A large randomized clinical trial has reported a potential interaction between CCB and statin in coronary heart disease. The dual treatment has also found to reduce statistically significant stroke incidence by 27%. It is suggested that the interaction between CCB and statin could lead to increased stability of atherosclerotic plaques [89].

However, well designed trials of coadministered CCB and statin in elderly hypertensive patients with or without cognitive dysfunction are not yet available.

Obviously, such trials are required to evaluate the clinical benefit of the combination of both CCB and statin in patients with VCI.

The plausible interactions between dihydropyridine CCBs and statins are shown in Figure 1.

Higher adherence to a Mediterranean- type dietary pattern, associated with slower cognitive decline in several observational studies, has been recommended for patients with cognitive impairment [24].

A recent multicentre randomized primary prevention trial, including 522 participants at high vascular risk, has also shown a beneficial effect of the Mediterranean diet on cognitive functions, that could be explained by its antioxidant and anti-inflammatory actions. The global cognitive performance has been evaluated by MMSE and Clock Drawing Test before and after 6.5 years of nutritional intervention [90].

Evidently, new larger controlled studies are needed to confirm the potential beneficial effects of the Mediterranean diet on cognitive functions in persons at high cerebrovascular risk.

As cerebral WMLs have often been found in elderly persons with long-standing poorly controlled hypertension, their protection should also be considered. The white matter, not only neurons, may be a target for innovative treatment approaches intended to improve functional recovery after its damage. In preclinical studies, different agents have been reported to attenuate the ischemic lesions of cerebral white matter [91–93]. However, these data have not been confirmed in clinical trials and MRI investigations.

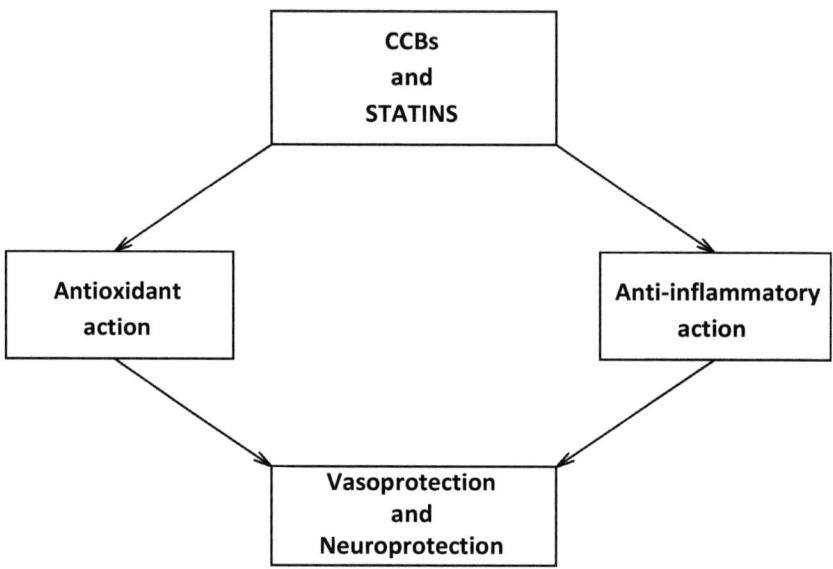

Figure 1. The antioxidant and anti-inflammatory actions of dihydropyridine CCBs and statins could lead to vasoprotection, including stability of atherosclerotic plaques, and to neuroprotection.

The treatment of the other concomitant VRFs, i.e. DM, hypercholesterolemia and heart disease, could reduce the risk of vascular cognitive disorders and delay the cognitive decline [94]. Undoubtedly, in elderly hypertensive patients multimodal interventions should be undertaken in the early stages of the vascular cognitive dysfunctions, prior to the occurrence of severe irreversible brain ischemic lesions with consequent VaD [95].

Discussion

The controversial results from the clinical trials on the effect of antihypertensive treatment in preventing or slowing dawn cognitive decline in elderly hypertensive persons indicate that further well designed studies are needed. .

Available data suggest that BP lowering in elderly patients with long-standing hypertension and cerebral small vessel disease below a certain critical level may decrease the blood flow in the deep subcortical structures and cause ischemic brain lesions, i.e. lacunes and/or leucoaraiosis with relevant clinical manifestations – impairment of attention and frontal lobe executive functions.

However, the threshold beyond which BP lowering may have deleterious effects needs to be determined [8]. Probably, it is not equal to all cases and may depend on different VRF. It has been pointed out that the recommendation of the guidelines to lower the SBP below 140 mm Hg also in elderly patients is not evidence-based **[96].** Recently, new hypertension guidelines, containing certain disagreements, have recommended a treatment threshold of 150 mm Hg SBP to patients 80 years or older but also to patients 60 years or older [97, 98].

On the other hand, it is established that the central BP, aortic or carotid, is different from the brachial BP and it is more closely related to the pathophysiology of the end-organ damage [99]. In chronically treated hypertensive patients, the carotid SBP is lower than the corresponding brachial SBP [100]. Apart from this, it has been suggested that the BP in patients with occlusive or severe stenotic diseases of the carotid or vertebral arteries should not be lowered excessively [101].

Recently, in a comprehensive scientific statement the evidence on vascular contribution to cognitive impairment and dementia has been reviewed. The dysfunction of neurovascular unit and mechanisms, regulating CBF are suggested to play an important role in the pathophysiology of VCI. The risk factors for VCI include hypertension, atrial fibrillation, DM, hypercholesterolemia and carotid intimal-medial thickness. The same risk factors may be also risk markers for Alzheimer disease. It is also pointed out that the role of hypertension in later life is not consistent and the issue of blood pressure treatment in older people remains open [24].

Obviously, the clinical criteria and the cerebral hemodynamics changes should be taken into account, considering the level of BP reduction in elderly persons. Repeated neuropsychological assessments, using appropriate standardized tests to identify persons in the early stages of cognitive impairment [102], are needed when antihypertensive treatment is carried out. The occurrence of subcortical-frontal cognitive impairments, even mild, requires proceeding to BP lowering with caution. In addition, the high-grade carotid stenoses and impaired CBF autoregulation should be considered when administering antihypertensive treatment to elderly subjects. TDS has proven to be an useful and most widely adopted method in the assessment of cerebral hemodynamics and the effects of different antihypertensive drugs. It is also relatively inexpensive [103–106]. TDS could become a valuable tool to monitor cerebral hemodynamics changes in elderly patients at high risk for cognitive decline with the aim to individualize the antihypertensive treatment and prevent further cerebral hypoperfusion [107].

In elderly hypertensive patients multimodal interventions, including neuroprotection, should be taken into consideration. It has been suggested that the blockade of the angiotensin-renin system may protect the brain against ischemia and cognitive decline. Dihydropyridine calcium channel blockers also claim neuroprotection. It seems that the combination of the angiotensin-renin system blockade or of a calcium channel blocker with statins may contribute to slow down the cognitive decline in elderly hypertensive patients. A Mediterranean- type dietary pattern, has been also recommended for patients with cognitive impairment The therapeutic approaches to the prevention of cerebral WMLs are future challenges.

Evidently, an appropriate and well controlled BP management and neuropotection in patients with VCI may prevent or postpone development of VaD.

Conclusion

Hypertension is an important modifiable risk factor for VCI and VaD. Antihypertensive therapy reduces the risk of cardiovascular morbidity and mortality. However, its role in preventing cognitive disorders in elderly hypertensive subjects without a history of stroke is still a matter of debate. Several studies have found cerebral WMLs on MRI in the majority of patients with long-standing and poorly controlled hypertension. The MRI changes have been shown to correlate with vascular cognitive disorders, particularly impairments of attention and executive function. In addition, it has been reported that excessive BP lowering in elderly persons could increase the risk of cerebral WMLs and of consequent vascular cognitive disorders. As a result of cerebral small vessel lesions in long-standing hypertension, CBF autoregulation is disrupted and excessive BP lowering may lead to further cerebral hypoperfusion and worsening of cognitive impairments. This is why the antihypertensive treatment in these cases should be based on the pathogenesis of the cognitive impairments, considering cerebral small vessel disease and high-grade carotid stenoses or occlusion. As perfusion magnetic resonance imaging is not widely available to demonstrate WMLs in elderly hypertensive patients, the individual clinical criteria, neuropsychological assessments, using appropriate standardized neuropsychological tests, and ultrasonography could be considered.

Cognitive functions, carotid artery disease and impaired CBF autoregulation should be taken into account when administering antihypertensive treatment to elderly subjects.

TDS has proven to be a useful method in the assessment of cerebral hemodynamics and the effects of antihypertensive drugs. The repeated neuropsychological assessments and ultrasonography to monitor cerebral hemodynamics changes in the course of antihypertensive treatment may decrease the risk of cerebral hypoperfusion and prevent or slow down cognitive decline in elderly hypertensive patients. A neuoprotection may be also taken into consideration. Prospective studies are needed to assess the benefit from such a treatment strategy.

References

1. Cacciatore F, Abete P, Ferrara N, Paolisso G, Amato L, Canonico S, Maggi S, Varricchio M, Rengo F. The role of blood pressure in cognitive impairment in an elderly population. Osservatorio Geriatrico Campano Group. J Hypertens 1997;15:135–42.
2. Starr JM, Deary IJ, Inch S, Cross S, MacLennan WJ. Blood pressure and cognitive decline in healthy old people. J Hum Hypertens 1997;11:777–81.
3. Skoog I. Status of risk factors for vascular dementia. Neuroepidemiology 1998;17:2–9.

4. Harrington F, Saxby BK, McKeith IG, Wesnes K, Ford GA. Cognitive performance in hypertensive and normotensive older subjects. Hypertension 2000;36:1079–82.

5. Paglieri C, Bisbocci D, Amenta F, Veglio F. Arterial hypertension and cognitive deficit. Ann Ital Med Int 2004 ;19:163–70.

6. Chobanian AV, Bakris GL, Black HR, Cushman WC, Green LA, Izzo JL Jr, et al.; Joint National Committee on Prevention, Detection, Evaluation, and Treatment of High Blood Pressure. National Heart, Lung, and Blood Institute; National High Blood Pressure Education Program Coordinating Committee: Seventh report of the Joint National Committee on Prevention, Detection, Evaluation, and Treatment of High Blood Pressure. Hypertension 2003; 42:1206–52.

7. Mancia G, De Backer G, Dominiczak A, Cifkova R, Fagard R, Germano G, et al. Guidelines for the Management of Arterial Hypertension: The Task Force for the Management of Arterial Hypertension of the European Society of Hypertension (ESH) and of the European Society of Cardiology (ESC). J Hypertens. 2007; 25(6):1105–87.

8. Birns J, Markus H, Kalra L. Blood pressure reduction for vascular risk: is there a price to be paid? Stroke 2005; 36:1308–13.

9. Sacco RL, Adams R, Albers G, Alberts MJ, Benavente O, Furie K,, et al; American Heart Association; American Stroke Association Council on Stroke; Council on Cardiovascular Radiology and Intervention; American Academy of Neurology: Guidelines for prevention of stroke in patients with ischemic stroke or transient ischemic attack. Stroke 2006; 37:577–617.

10. Vasan RS, Larson MG, Leip EP, Kannel WB, Levy D. Assessment of frequency of progression to hypertension in non-hypertensive participants in the Framingham Heart Study: a cohort study. Lancet 2001; 358:1682–6.

11. Birns J, Morris R, Donaldson N, Kalra L. The effects of blood pressure reduction on cognitive function: a review of effects based on pooled data from clinical trials. J Hypertens. 2006;24(10):1907–14.

12. Guo Z, Fratiglioni L, Winblad B, Viitanen M. Blood pressure and performance on the Mini-Mental State Examination in the very old. Cross-sectional and longitudinal data from the Kungsholmen Project. Am J Epidemiol 1997; 145(12): 1106–13.

13. Nilsson SE, Read S, Berg S, Johansson B, Melander A, Lindblad U. Low systolic blood pressure is associated with impaired cognitive function in the oldest old: longitudinal observations in a population-based sample 80 years and older. Aging Clin Exp Res 2007; 19(1): 41–7.

14. Skoog I, Lernfelt B, Landahl S, Palmertz B, Andreasson LA, Nilsson L, Persson G, Oden A, Svanborg A.15-year longituidal study of blood pressure and dementia. Lancet 1996; 347(9009): 1141–5.

15. Launer LJ, Masaki K, Petrovitch H, Foley D, Havlik RJ. The association between midlife blood pressure levels and late-life cognitive function. The Honolulu-Asia Aging Study. JAMA 1995; 274(23): 1846–51.

16. Launer LJ, Ross GW, Petrovitch H, Masaki K, Foley D, White LR, Havlik RJ. Midlife blood pressure and dementia: the Honolulu–Asia aging study. Neurobiol Aging 2000; 21(1): 49–55.

17. Swan GE, DeCarli C, Miller BL, Reed T, Wolf PA, Jack LM, Carmelli D. Association of midlife blood pressure to late-life cognitive decline and brain morphology Neurology. 1998 Oct; 51(4): 986–93.

18. Swan GE, Carmelli D, Larue A. Systolic Blood Pressure Tracking Over 25 to 30 Years and Cognitive Performance in Older Adults. Stroke. 1998; 29 (11): 2334–40.

19. Kilander L, Nyman H, Boberg M, Hansson L, Lithell H. Hypertension is related to cognitive impairment: a 20-year follow-up of 999 men. Hypertension 1998; 31(3): 780–6.

20. Elias PK, Elias MF, Robbins MA, Budge MM. Blood pressure-related cognitive decline: does age make a difference? Hypertension. 2004;44(5):631–6.

21. Hebert LE, Scherr PA, Bennett DA, Bienias JL, Wilson RS, Morris MC, Evans DA. Blood pressure and late-life cognitive function change: a biracial longitudinal population study. Neurology 2004; 62(11): 2021–2024

22. . Ruitenberg A, den Heijer T, Bakker SL, van Swieten JC, Koudstaal PJ, Hofman A, Breteler MM. Cerebral hypoperfusion and clinical onset of dementia: the Rotterdam Study. Ann Neurol 2005; 57(6): 789–794

23. Vera-Cuesta H, Vera-Acosta H, Leon-Benito O, Fernandez-Maderos I. Prevalence and risk factors of age-related memory disorder in a health district. Rev Neurol 2006; 43(3): 137–142.

24. Gorelick PB, Scuteri A, Black SE, Decarli C, Greenberg SM, Iadecola C, Launer LJ, Laurent S, Lopez OL, Nyenhuis D, Petersen RC, Schneider JA, Tzourio C, Arnett DK, Bennett DA, Chui HC, Higashida RT, Lindquist R, Nilsson PM, Roman GC, Sellke FW, Seshadri S; Vascular contributions to cognitive impairment and dementia: a statement for healthcare professionals from the american heart association/american stroke association. Stroke. 2011; 42:2672–713.

25. Strandgaard S. Autoregulation of cerebral blood flow in hypertensive patients. The modifying influence of prolonged antihypertensive treatment

on the tolerance to acute, drug-induced hypotension. Strandgaard S. Circulation. 1976; 53(4):720–7.

26. Barry DI. Cerebral blood flow in hypertension. J Cardiovasc Pharmacol 1985; 7 (Suppl 2):S94–8.

27. Barry DI. Cerebrovascular aspects of antihypertensive treatment. Am J Cardiol 1989; 63:14C–8C.

28. Meyer JS, Rogers RL, Mortel KF. Prospective analysis of long term control of mild hypertension on cerebral blood flow. Stroke 1985; 16:985–90.

29. Rodriguez G, Arvigo F, Marenco S, Nobili F, Romano P, Sandini G, Rosadini G. Regional cerebral blood flow in essential hypertension: data evaluation by a mapping system. Stroke 1987; 18:13–20.

30. Nobili F, Rodriguez G, Marenco S, De Carli F, Gambaro M, Castello C, et al. Regional cerebral blood flow in chronic hypertension. A correlative study. Stroke 1993; 24:1148–53.

31. Beason-Held LL, Moghekar A, Zonderman AB, Kraut MA, Resnick SM. Longitudinal changes in cerebral blood flow in the older hypertensive brain. Stroke. 2007; 38:1766–73.

32. Mentis MJ, Salerno J, Horwitz B, Grady C, Schapiro MB, Murphy DG, Rapoport SI. Reduction of functional neuronal connectivity in long-term treated hypertension. Stroke 1994; 25:601–7.

33. Salerno JA, Grady C, Mentis M, Gonzalez-Aviles A, Wagner E, Schapiro MB, Rapoport SI. Brain metabolic function in older men with chronic essential hypertension. J Gerontol A Biol Sci Med Sci 1995; 50:M147–54.

34. Sierra C, de la Sierra A, Chamorro A, Larrousse M, Domenech M, Coca A. Cerebral hemodynamics and silent cerebral white matter lesions in middle-aged essential hypertensive patients. Blood Press 2004; 13):304–9.

35. Zhang P, Huang Y, Li Y, Lu M, Wu Y. A large-scale study on relationship between cerebral blood flow velocity and blood pressure in a natural population. J Hum Hypertens 2006; 20:742–8.

36. Hougaku H, Matsumoto M, Kitagawa K, Harada K, Oku N, Itoh T, et al. Silent cerebral infarction as a form of hypertensive target organ damage in the brain. Hypertension 1992; 20:816–20.

37. Schmidt R, Fazekas F, Koch M, Kapeller P, Augustin M, Offenbacher H, et al. Magnetic resonance imaging cerebral abnormalities and neuropsychologic test performance in elderly hypertensive subjects. A case-control study. Arch Neurol 1995; 52:905–10.

38. Strassburger TL, Lee HC, Daly EM, Szczepanik J, Krasuski JS, Mentis MJ, et al. Interactive effects of age and hypertension on volumes of brain structures. Stroke 1997; 28:1410–17.

39. O'Brien JT, Wiseman R, Burton EJ, Barber B, Wesnes K, Saxby B, Ford GA. Cognitive associations of subcortical white matter lesions in older people. Ann N Y Acad Sci 2002; 977:436–44.

40. Heijer T, Skoog I, Oudkerk M, de Leeuw FE, de Groot JC, Hofman A, Breteler MM. Association between blood pressure levels over time and brain atrophy in the elderly. Neurobiol Aging 2003; 24:307–13.

41. van Dijk EJ, Breteler MM, Schmidt R, Berger K, Nilsson LG, Oudkerk M, et al; CASCADE Consortium: The association between blood pressure, hypertension, and cerebral white matter lesions: cardiovascular determinants of dementia study. Hypertension 2004; 44:625–30.

42. Wiseman RM, Saxby BK, Burton EJ, Barber R, Ford GA, O'Brien JT. Hippocampal atrophy, whole brain volume, and white matter lesions in older hypertensive subjects. Neurology 2004; 63:1892–7.

43. Verghese J, Lipton RB, Hall CB, Kuslansky G, Katz MJ. Low blood pressure and the risk of dementia in very old individuals. Neurology 2003; 61:1667–72.

44. Qiu C, von Strauss E, Fastbom J, Winblad B, Fratiglioni L. Low blood pressure and risk of dementia in the Kungsholmen project: a 6-year follow-up study. Arch Neurol 2003; 60:223–8.

45. Qiu C, von Strauss E, Winblad B, Fratiglioni L. Decline in blood pressure over time and risk of dementia: a longitudinal study from the Kungsholmen project. Stroke. 2004; 35:1810–5.

46. Nilsson SE, Read S, Berg S, Johansson B, Melander A, Lindblad U. Low systolic blood pressure is associated with impaired cognitive function in the oldest old: longitudinal observations in a population-based sample 80 years and older. Aging Clin Exp Res. 2007; 19:41–7.

47. O'Brien JT, Erkinjuntti T, Reisberg B, Roman G, Sawada T, Pantoni L, et al. Vascular cognitive impairment. Lancet Neurol 2003; 2: 89–98.

48. O'Brien JT. Vascular cognitive impairment. Am J Geriatr Psychiatry 2006; 14: 724–33.

49. Kannel WB. Risk stratification in hypertension: new insights from the Framingham Study. Am J Hypertens 2000; 13:3S–10S.

50. Foucan L, Bangou-Bredent J, Ekouevi DK, Deloumeaux J, Roset JE, Kangambega P. Hypertension and combinations of cardiovascular risk factors. An epidemiologic casecontrol study in an adult population in Guadeloupe (FWI).Eur J Epidemiol 2001; 17:1089–95.

51. Hadjiev DI, Mineva PP, Vukov MI. Multiple modifiable risk factors for first ischemic stroke: a population-based epidemiological study. Eur J Neurol 2003; 10:577–82.

52. Schmidt R, Fazekas F, Kleinert G, Offenbacher H, Gindl K, Payer F, et al. Magnetic resonance imaging signal hyperintensities in the deep and subcortical white matter. A comparative study between stroke patients and normal volunteers. Arch Neurol 1992; 49:825–7.

53. O'Leary DH, Polak JF, Kronmal RA, Kittner SJ, Bond MG, Wolfson SK Jr, et al. Distribution and correlates of sonographically detected carotid artery disease in the Cardiovascular Health Study. The CHS Collaborative Research Group. Stroke 1992; 23:1752–60.

54. Fine-Edelstein JS, Wolf PA, O'Leary DH, Poehlman H, Belanger AJ, Kase CS, D'Agostino RB. Precursors of extracranial carotid atherosclerosis in the Framingham Study. Neurology 1994; 44:1046–50.

55. Mannami T, Konishi M, Baba S, Nishi N, Terao A. Prevalence of asymptomatic carotid atherosclerosis lesions detected by high - resolution ultrasonography and its relation to cardiovascular risk factors in the general population of a Japanese city: the Suita Study. Stroke 1997; 28:518–25.

56. Rao R. The role of carotid stenosis in vascular cognitive impairment. J Neurol Sci 2002; 203-204:103–7.

57. Johnston SC, O'Meara ES, Manolio TA, Lefkowitz D, O'Leary DH, Goldstein S, et al. Cognitive impairment and decline are associated with carotid artery disease in patients without clinically evident cerebrovascular disease. Ann Intern Med 2004; 140:237–47.

58. Mathiesen EB, Waterloo K, Joakimsen O, Bakke SJ, Jacobsen EA, Bonaa KH. Reduced neuropsychological test performance in asymptomatic carotid stenosis: The Tromso Study. Neurology 2004; 62:695–701.

59. Foucan L, Bangou-Bredent J, Ekouevi DK, Deloumeaux J, Roset JE, Kangambega P. Hypertension and combinations of cardiovascular risk

factors. An epidemiologic case-control study in an adult population in Guadeloupe (FWI). Eur J Epidemiol 2001; 17(12):1089–95.

60. Boden-Albala BM, Lee HS, Paik MC, Giardina E, Rundek T, Sacco RL. Stroke risk and the metabolic syndrome: findings from the Northern Manhattan Study. American Academy of Neurology, 55th Annual Meeting, March 29 – April 5, 2003 Honolulu, Hawaii, S33.001.

61. Bowler JV, Gorelick PB. Advances in vascular cognitive impairment 2006.Stroke. 2007; 38(2):241–4.

62. Hadjiev DI, Mineva PP. Antihypertensive treatment in elderly hypertensives without a history of stroke and the risk of cognitive disorders.Acta Neurol Scand. 2008 ; 118(3):139–45.

63. Wiederkehr S, Laurin D, Simard M, Verreault R, Lindsay J.Vascular risk factors and cognitive functions in nondemented elderly individuals. J Geriatr Psychiatry Neurol. 2009 Sep;22(3):196–206.

64. SHEP Cooperative Research Group. Prevention of stroke by antihypertensive drug treatment in older persons with isolated systolic hypertension. JAMA 1991; 265: 3255–64.

65. Prince MJ, Bird AS, Blizard RA, Mann AH. Is the cognitive function of older patients affected by antihypertensive treatment? Results from 54 months of the medical research council's trial of hypertension in older adults. BMJ 1996; 30,312: 801–5.

66. Forette F, Seux ML, Staessen JA, Thijs L, Birkenhäger WH, Babarskiene MR, et al. Prevention of dementia in randomized double-blind placebo-controlled systolic Hypertension in Europe (Syst-Eur) trial. Lancet 1998; 352:1347–51.

67. Lithell H, Hansson L, Skoog I, Elmfeldt D, Hofman A, Olofsson B, et al.; SCOPE Study Group. The study on cognition and prognosis in the elderly

(SCOPE): principal results of a randomized double-blind intervention trial. J Hypertens 2003; 21(5): 875–6.

68. Skoog I, Lithell H, Hansson L, Elmfeldt D, Hofman A, Olofsson B, et al.; SCOPE Study Group. Effect of baseline cognitive function and antihypertensive treatment on cognitive and cardiovascular outcomes: study on COgnition and prognosis in the elderly (SCOPE). Am J Hypertens 2005; 18(8): 1052–9.

69. Peters R, Beckett N, Forette F, Tuomilehto J, Clarke R, Ritchie C, et al.; HYVET investigators. Incident dementia and blood pressure lowering in the Hypertension in the Very Elderly Trial cognitive function assessment (HYVET-COG): a double-blind, placebo controlled trial. Lancet Neurol. 2008; 7(8):683–9.

70. McGuinness B, Todd S, Passmore P, Bullock R. Blood pressure lowering in patients without prior cerebrovascular disease for prevention of cognitive impairment and dementia. Cochrane Database Syst Rev 2009; (4):CD004–CD034.

71. Waldstein SR, Giggey PP, Thayer JF, Zonderman AB. Nonlinear relations of blood pressure to cognitive function: the Baltimore Longitudinal Study of Aging. Hypertension 2005; 45(3): 374–9.

72. Hadjiev D, Mineva P. Antihypertensive Treatment in Reducing the Risk of Dementia. Stroke 2006; 37:2869.

73. Thybo NK, Stephens N, Cooper A, Aalkjaer C, Heagerty AM, Mulvany MJ. Effect of antihypertensive treatment on small arteries of patients with previously untreated essential hypertension. Hypertension 1995; 25: 474–81.

74. Baumbach GL, Chillon JM. Effects of angiotensin-converting enzyme inhibitors on cerebral vascular structure in chronic hypertension. J Hypertens 2000; 18(1): Suppl, 7–11.

75. Chillon JM, Baumbach GL. Effects of an angiotensin-converting enzyme inhibitor and a beta-blocker on cerebral arteriolar dilatation in hypertensive rats. Hypertension 2001; 37(6): 1388–93.

76. Fournier A, Achard JM, Boutitie F, Mazouz H, Mansour J, Oprisiu R, Fernandez L, Messerli F. Is the angiotensin II Type 2 receptor cerebroprotective? Curr Hypertens Rep 2004; 6(3): 182–9.

77. Fournier A, Messerli FH, Achard JM, Fernandez L. Cerebroprotection mediated by angiotensin II: a hypothesis supported by recent randomized clinical trials. J Am Coll Cardiol 2004; 43(8): 1343–7.

78. Schrader J, Luders S, Kulschewski A, Hammersen F, Plate K, Berger J, Zidek W, Dominiak P, Diener HC; MOSES Study Group. Morbidity and Mortality After Stroke, Eprosartan Compared with Nitrendipine for Secondary Prevention: principal results of a prospective randomized controlled study (MOSES). Stroke 2005; 36: 1218–26.

79. Das UN. Is angiotensin II an endogenious pro-inflamatory molecule? Med Sci Monit 2005; 11(5): RA155–62.

80. Fogari R, Zoppi A. Effect of antihypertensive agents on quality of life in the elderly. Drugs Aging 2004; 21(6): 377–93.

81. Inzitari D, Poggesi A. Calcium channel blockers and stroke. Aging Clin Exp Res 2005; 17(4 Suppl): 16–30.

82. Verdecchia P, Reboldi G, Angeli F, Gattobigio R, Bentivoglio M, Thijs L, Staessen JA, Porcellati C. Angiotensin-converting enzyme inhibitors and calcium channel blockers for coronary heart disease and stroke prevention. Hypertension 2005; 46(2): 386–92.

83. Hanon O, Pequignot R, Seux ML, Lenoir H, Bune A, Rigaud AS, Forette F, Girerd X. Relationship between antihypertensive drug therapy and

cognitive function in elderly hypertensive patients with memory complaints. J Hypertens. 2006; 24(10):2101–7.

84. Vaughan CJ, Delanty N. Neuroprotective properties of statins in cerebral ischemia and stroke. Stroke 1999; 30: 1969–73.

85. Vaughan GJ. Prevention of stroke with statins: Effects beyond lipid lowering. The Am J Cardiol 2003; 91: 23B–29B.

86. Zacco A, Togo J, Spence K, Ellis A, Lloyd D, Furlong S, Piser T. 3-hydroxy-3-methylglutaryl coenzyme A reductase inhibitors protect cortical neurons from excitotoxicity. J Neurosci 2003; 23: 11104–11.

87. Bosel J, Gandor F, Harms C, Synowitz M, Harms U, Djoufack PC, Megow D, Dirnagl U, Hortnagl H, Fink KB, Endres M. Neuroprotective effects atorvastatin against glotamate-induced excitotoxicity in primary cortical neurons. J Neurochem 2005; 92: 1386–98.

88. Kumar S, Savitz S, Schlaug G, Caplan L, Selim M. Antiplatelets, ACE inhibitors, and statins combination reduces stroke severity and tissue at risk. Neurology 2006; 66: 1153–8.

89. Sever P, Dahlöf B, Poulter N, Wedel H, Beevers G, Caulfield M, Collins R, Kjeldsen S, Kristinsson A, McInnes G, Mehlsen J, Nieminem M, O'Brien E, Ostergren J; ASCOT Steering Committee Members. Potential synergy between lipid-lowering and blood-pressure-lowering in the Anglo-Scandinavian Cardiac Outcomes Trial. Eur Heart J. 2006 Dec;27 (24):2982–8

90. Martínez-Lapiscina EH, Clavero P, Toledo E, Estruch R, Salas-Salvadó J, San Julián B, Sanchez-Tainta A, Ros E, Valls-Pedret C, Martinez-Gonzalez MÁ. Mediterranean diet improves cognition: the PREDIMED-NAVARRA randomised trial. J Neurol Neurosurg Psychiatry. 2013; 84(12):1318–25.

91. Follett PL, Rosenberg PA, Volpe JJ, Jensen FE. NBQX attenuates excitotoxic injury in developing white matter. J Neurosci 2000; 20(24): 9235–41.

92. Goldberg MP, Ransom BR. New light on white matter. Stroke 2003; 34: 330–2.

93. Follett PL, Deng W, Dai W, Talos DM, Massillon LJ, Rosenberg PA, Volpe JJ, Jensen FE. Glutamate receptor-mediated oligodendrocyte toxicity in periventricular leukomalacia: a protective role for topiramate. J Neurosci 2004; 24(18): 4412–20.

94. Martinez-Vila E, Murie-Fernandez M, Gallego Perez-Larraya J, Irimia P. Neuroprotection in vascular dementia. Cerebrovasc Dis 2006; 21 Suppl 2: 106–7.

95. Hadjiev D, Mineva P. Hypertension, vascular cognitive disorders and neuroprotection. Acta Neuropsychiatrica 2007: 19: 269–78.

96. Zanchetti A, Grassi G, Mancia G. When should antihypertensive drug treatment be initiated and to what levels should systolic blood pressure be lowered? A critical reappraisal. J Hypertens. 2009; 27(5):923–34.

97. Mancia G, Fagard R, Narkiewicz K, Redon J, Zanchetti A, Böhm M, Christiaens T, Cifkova R, De Backer G, Dominiczak A, Galderisi M, Grobbee DE, Jaarsma T, Kirchhof P, Kjeldsen SE, Laurent S, Manolis AJ, Nilsson PM, Ruilope LM, Schmieder RE, Sirnes PA, Sleight P, Viigimaa M, Waeber B, Zannad F. 2013 ESH/ESC Practice Guidelines for the Management of Arterial Hypertension.Blood Press. 2013 Dec 20. [Epub ahead of print]

98. James PA, Oparil S, Carter BL, Cushman WC, Dennison-Himmelfarb C, Handler J, Lackland DT, Lefevre ML, Mackenzie TD, Ogedegbe O, Smith SC Jr, Svetkey LP, Taler SJ, Townsend RR, Wright JT Jr, Narva AS, Ortiz

E. 2014 Evidence-Based Guideline for the Management of High Blood Pressure in Adults: Report From the Panel Members Appointed to the Eighth Joint National Committee (JNC 8). JAMA. 2013 Dec 18.. [Epub ahead of print]

99. Protogerou AD, Papaioannou TG, Blacher J, Papamichael CM, Lekakis JP, Safar ME. Central blood pressures: do we need them in the management of cardiovascular disease? Is it a feasible therapeutic target? J Hypertens. 2007; 25(2):265–72.

100.Safar ME, Blacher J, Protogerou A, Achimastos A. Arterial stiffness and central hemodynamics in treated hypertensive subjects according to brachial blood pressure classification. J Hypertens. 2008; 26(1):130–7.

101.European Stroke Initiative Executive Committee; EUSI Writing Committee, Olsen TS, Langhorne P, Diener HC, Hennerici M, Ferro J, Sivenius J, et al. European stroke initiative recommendations for stroke management – update 2003. Cerebrovasc Dis 2003; 16:311–37.

102.Hachinski V, Iadecola C, Petersen RC, Breteler MM, Nyenhuis DL, Black SE, et al. National Institute of Neurological Disorders and Stroke-Canadian Stroke Network vascular cognitive impairment harmonization standards. Stroke. 2006; 37:2220–41.

103.Troisi E, Attanasio A, Matteis M, Bragoni M, Monaldo BC, Caltagirone C, Silvestrini M. Cerebral hemodynamics in young hypertensive subjects and effects of atenolol treatment. J Neurol Sci. 1998; 159(1):115–9.

104.Walters M, Muir S, Shah I, Lees K. Effect of perindopril on cerebral vasomotor reactivity in patients with lacunar infarction. Stroke. 2004; 35(8):1899–902.

105.Fu CH, Yang CC, Kuo TB. Effects of different classes of antihypertensive drugs on cerebral hemodynamics in elderly hypertensive patients. Am J Hypertens 2005; 18:1621–25.

106.Yam AT, Lang EW, Lagopoulos J, Yip K, Griffith J, Mudaliar Y, Dorsch NW. Cerebral autoregulation and ageing. J Clin Neurosci. 2005; 12(6):643–46.

107.Hadjiev DI, Mineva PP. Antihypertensive treatment with cerebral hemodynamics monitoring by ultrasonography in elderly hypertensives without a history of stroke may prevent or slow down cognitive decline. A pending issue. Med Hypotheses. 2011; 76(3):434–7.

Acknowledgement

The author wish to express his appreciation to Philip B. Gorelick, MD MPH FACP FAAN FANA FAHA Professor, Translational Science and Molecular Medicine, Michigan State University College of Human Medicine; Medical Director, Mercy Health Hauenstein Neurosciences, Grand Rapids, Michigan for his helpful suggestions.

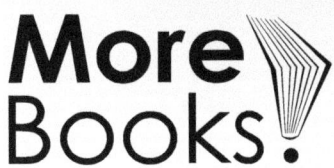
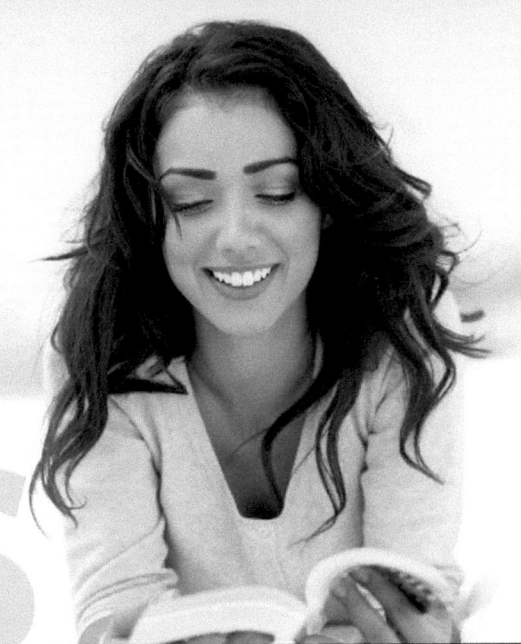
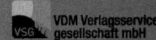

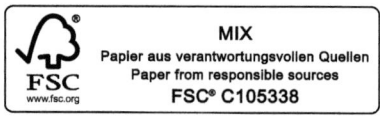